# Chair Yoga for Seniors Over 60

**Step by step guide with gentle exercises to live happily in pain free, and improve mobility, balance, strength and flexibility with 15-minutes daily routine challenge**

By

## Ellie M. Nelson

# TABLE OF CONTENTS

# Introduction

In the tapestry of life, as we age gracefully, we often find ourselves facing new challenges and exploring different paths to happiness.

One of these paths, perhaps less traveled but extremely rewarding, is chair yoga.

This unique practice is a gentle, holistic, and rejuvenating journey that invites seniors over 60 to embrace the art of wellness with open arms and open hearts.

As we enter our golden years, the idea of starting a rigorous exercise routine can seem intimidating.

However, the benefits of an active lifestyle are undeniable. This is where chair yoga shines as a beacon of hope. It's a practice that offers all the benefits of traditional yoga but is specifically designed for those of us who like or need the support of a chair.

# Why chair yoga for seniors?

Chair yoga is more than just a modified version of yoga; it is a bridge to a world full of vitality and peace, regardless of your age or physical condition. It recognizes the wisdom your body has accumulated over decades and seeks to honor and nurture it.

Here's why chair yoga is great for people over 60:

**Accessibility:** The chair becomes a solid support for you, allowing you to practice yoga without having to worry about your complicated and uncomfortable posture. It's the ultimate equalizer, inclusive of all body types and abilities.

**Safety first:** One of the biggest concerns as we age is safety. With chair yoga, you can practice comfortably without fear of slipping or falling, making it the safest choice for senior fitness.

**Gentle yet effective:** The yoga chair may be gentle yet effective. It provides an avenue to improve flexibility, balance, strength, and mental clarity while being gentle on the joints.

**Mental health:** As we age, mental health is just as important as physical health. Chair yoga integrates mindfulness and meditation, promoting mental clarity and emotional well-being.

**Community:** chair yoga classes often provide a sense of community, an opportunity to connect with others on similar journeys. These connections can be just as valuable as the material benefits.

## What to expect in this journey?

Over the next 30 days, we will embark on a remarkable adventure of self-discovery and transformation.

Together we will explore a complete program that will introduce you to the world of chair yoga.

We will start slowly, building a solid foundation, and gradually progress to more advanced practices. Each day, you'll experience a 15-minute chair yoga routine designed to improve flexibility, balance, and overall health.

This book is more than just a manual; it is your companion. It will guide you through poses, Breathwork, and meditation practices to make chair yoga an enriching experience. You will discover the power of breathing, the grace of movement, and peace of mind.

Additionally, we'll provide you with a 30-day meal plan designed to complement your chair yoga practice. A good diet is the foundation of good health and when you practice chair yoga, we want to make sure your body is getting the nutrients it needs.


So, dear reader, whether you are new to yoga, have some experience, have physical limitations, or are simply looking for a gentle approach to wellness, chair yoga may be the guide for you.

It is an invitation to live an active, balanced, and fulfilling life for the best years to come.

Join us on this transformative journey and explore together the world of chair yoga for seniors over 60 years old.


***********************************************


Welcome to a transformative journey that celebrates the vitality and happiness of seniors over the age of 60.

In this comprehensive guide, we'll explore the world of chair yoga, a practice designed to empower, strengthen, and rejuvenate.

This chapter is our starting point for a deeper dive into the importance of yoga for seniors, reveals the many benefits of chair yoga, and provides an overview of a 30-day plan that will guide you to a more balanced, healthier state and harmonious life. Together, let us embark on this path to happiness.

# Importance of Chair Yoga for Seniors

As we age gracefully, life brings us countless experiences and abundant wisdom. However, it also poses unique challenges to our physical and mental health.

Taking a holistic approach to health is important, and chair yoga is a powerful ally for seniors.

**Physical Resilience:** Chair Yoga with its gentle but effective method helps us maintain physical vitality. It promotes strength, flexibility, and balance, which is especially valuable as we age. These benefits not only prevent stiffness and discomfort in joints and muscles but also help us stay agile and active.

**Mental Clarity and Emotional Well-being:** Beyond the physical aspect, chair yoga also provides a serene haven for mental clarity and emotional balance. Stress reduction, mindful breathing, and meditation practices are integral parts of chair yoga, which are powerful tools for navigating the emotional and psychological aspects of aging.

**Preventive Health:** Regular yoga practice has been linked to preventing chronic diseases that often appear with age, including heart disease, diabetes, and osteoporosis. Chair Yoga supports circulation, strengthens the immune system, and improves digestion.

**Stress Relief:** Chair Yoga acts as a refuge from the chaos of daily life. It is a place to let go, relax, and find peace. Through its therapeutic approach, yoga helps reduce stress and anxiety and brings a deep sense of calm.

# Benefits of Chair Yoga for Seniors

Chair yoga, a variation of traditional yoga, is a training method especially suitable for people over 60 years old, bringing countless benefits.

**Accessibility:** Chair yoga is an inclusive practice that welcomes people of all physical conditions and all levels of yoga experience. The chair serves as a reliable accessory, providing stability and reducing the risk of injury.

**Improve Agility:** Over the next 30 days, you'll embark on a journey to improve agility. This newfound flexibility enhances comfort in everyday movements and reduces discomfort associated with stiffness.

**Improve Balance:** Aging can often lead to balance problems. Chair yoga is structured to address these concerns, incorporating exercises and poses designed to improve stability and reduce the risk of falls.

**Strength and Endurance:** Chair Yoga focuses on gradually developing strength and endurance, making daily activities easier. Stronger muscles also reduce joint discomfort.

**Mindfulness and Relaxation:** The practice integrates mindfulness and meditation techniques, reducing stress and promoting mental clarity and emotional well-being. This promotes a feeling of inner peace and contentment.

# 30-Day Plan Overview

At the heart of this journey is a comprehensive 30-day plan.

Over the next month, we'll be embarking on a carefully curated exploration of chair yoga. Each day, you'll experience a 15-minute chair yoga routine designed to improve your flexibility, balance, and overall health.
Our plan is a structured and progressive journey. We will start with basic practices and gradually progress to more complex poses and sequences.

Whether you are new to yoga or have previous yoga experience, our step-by-step guide will make it easier for you.

To complement your Chair Yoga practice, we have included a 30-day meal plan that ensures your body receives the nourishment it needs for optimal health. Nutrition is a cornerstone of well-being, and we aim to help you achieve balance in body and mind.

# Chapter 1

## Week 1: Getting Started with Chair Yoga for Seniors Over 60

As we age, maintaining our physical and mental health becomes more and more important.

For adults over 60, this often means looking for low-impact exercise options that are gentle on the body but still effective.

Chair yoga is one option that has gained popularity due to its adaptability and accessibility.

In this comprehensive guide, we'll begin your first week of chair yoga for seniors over 60.

We will explore daily routines, exercises, and relaxation techniques specifically designed to enhance the health and well-being of older adults.

The goal of this chapter is to provide a solid foundation for your chair yoga practice and set the stage for the weeks ahead.

# Day 1-5:  Introduction to Chair Yoga

Before diving into the specifics of chair yoga exercises and routines, it is essential to understand what chair yoga is and Why is it especially suitable for people over 60 years old.

**What is Chair Yoga?**

Chair yoga is a gentle form of yoga that is practiced while sitting on a chair or using a chair for support. It is designed to make yoga accessible to individuals with various physical limitations, including seniors, those recovering from injuries, or people with mobility issues.

Chair yoga adapts traditional yoga poses and exercises to be performed in a seated or supported position.

# Benefits of Chair Yoga for Seniors Over 60

**Improved Flexibility:** Chair yoga helps to improve joint mobility and flexibility, making daily activities easier and reducing the risk of injury.

**Enhanced Strength:** Engaging in chair yoga exercises strengthens the muscles that support the body, which is crucial for maintaining balance and preventing falls.

**Better Posture:** Practicing chair yoga encourages proper alignment and posture, which can reduce back pain and improve overall body mechanics.

**Stress Reduction:** The mindful breathing and relaxation techniques of chair yoga promote mental calmness and reduce stress and anxiety.

**Pain Management:** Chair yoga can be an effective way to manage chronic pain, such as arthritis or lower back pain.

**Community and social connection:** group chair yoga classes allow older adults to socialize, reducing feelings of isolation and loneliness.

**Increased Body Awareness:** Chair yoga helps older adults become more aware of their bodies, allowing them to notice and manage physical discomfort or imbalances sooner.

# Getting Started

Before you begin your chair yoga journey, here are some tips to keep in mind:

**Consult your healthcare professional:** If you have any underlying health condition or concern, it is essential to consult your healthcare professional before starting a new exercise routine.

**Choose the right chair:** Choose a sturdy armless chair with a flat, sturdy seat.
 Make sure it doesn't slide easily and is at the right height so you can sit comfortably with your feet flat on the floor.

**Dress comfortably:** Wear loose, breathable clothing that allows you to move freely.
 Comfortable shoes are also essential.

**Create a private space:** Find a quiet, well-lit place where you can set up a chair and practice chair yoga without distractions.

**Listen to your body:** Chair yoga includes gentle movements and stretches.

It's important to respect your body's limits and not subject yourself to discomfort or pain.

Now that you understand the basics of chair yoga, let's move on to the basics of the first week of practice.

# Breath Awareness and Relaxation

Breathing is a fundamental aspect of yoga, and it plays a significant role in chair yoga, especially when it comes to relaxation and mindfulness.

Proper breath awareness can help you manage stress and improve your overall sense of well-being.

The Importance of Breath Awareness In chair yoga, breath awareness is used to connect the mind and body, allowing you to focus on the present moment and relax.

Deep, controlled breathing can reduce stress, lower blood pressure, and help calm the nervous system.

### Day 1: Deep Breathing Exercises

On the first day of your chair yoga journey, start with a simple deep breathing exercise.
Here's how to do it:

- Sit comfortably on a chair, feet flat on the floor, hands on your knees.
- Close your eyes and take a moment to settle into a relaxing position.
- Inhale deeply through your nose, letting your belly expand as you fill your lungs.
- Exhale slowly and completely through your mouth.
- Continue this deep breathing pattern for 5 minutes.
- In this exercise, focus your attention on your breathing and let go of any distracting thoughts.

By breathing deeply and consciously, you can begin to feel relaxed and at peace.

**Day 2: Guided Relaxation Guided**

Relaxation is an effective way to reduce stress and promote mental and physical relaxation.
Find a quiet space, turn on some soothing music, and follow these relaxation instructions:

- Sit comfortably on a chair with your feet flat on the floor.
- Close your eyes and take a few deep breaths to center yourself.
- Imagine a peaceful place, such as a beach, forest, or garden.
- Imagine yourself there, paying attention to the sights, sounds, and feelings.
- As you breathe deeply, release tension with each exhalation.
 Feel the relaxation spread throughout your body.
- Spend 10-15 minutes relaxing with this guide to help you relax completely.

Guided relaxation is a great way to start chair yoga because it sets a peaceful tone and prepares you mentally for the physical exercises that follow.

## Day 3: Breath and Body Awareness

Integrate body awareness into breath practice to deepen the connection between breath and movement.

This exercise can also help you identify areas of tension in your body.

- Sit on a chair with your feet flat on the floor and your hands resting on your knees.
- Take a few deep breaths to relax.
- As you inhale, direct your attention to a specific area of your body, such as your shoulders.
- Imagine the breath flowing through this area and relaxing it.
- Exhale and release any tension from this area.
- Repeat this process, focusing on different parts of the body, including the neck, chest, arms, and legs.

This practice promotes relaxation and mindfulness, allowing you to become more aware of areas where you may feel stressed.

It is especially useful for older people who often suffer from joint stiffness in various parts of the body.

## Day 4: Breathing for Stress Relief

Breathing for Stress Relief is a technique that you can use in everyday life to manage stress and anxiety.

This can be especially beneficial for older adults, as stress can worsen many different health conditions.

- Sit on a chair, feet flat on the floor, hands on knees.
- Close your eyes and take a few deep breaths to center yourself.
- Breathe deeply for a count of four, letting your belly expand as you inhale.
- Hold your breath and count to four.
- Exhale slowly and completely to a count of six.
- Continue this 4-4-6 breathing pattern for 5-10 minutes.

This controlled breathing technique helps activate the body's relaxation response and reduce the "fight or flight" stress response.

It's an excellent tool for managing stress in any situation.

## Day 5: Combining Breath and Movement

On day five, combine breath awareness with gentle movements to prepare for the chair yoga exercises that follow.

This will help you synchronize your breathing with your body's movements, promoting feelings of mindfulness and presence.

- Sit on a chair with your feet flat on the floor and your hands resting on your knees.
- Inhale as you slowly raise your arms out in front of you, palms facing up.
- Exhale as you return your hands to your knees.
- Repeat this movement, synchronizing your breathing with the raising and lowering of your arms.

This simple exercise connects your breath to your movements, helping you stay present and focused.

This is a great way to move from relaxation to the active part of your chair yoga practice.

# Gentle Neck and Shoulders Stretches

The neck and shoulders are common areas of tension, especially in older adults, who may feel stiffness and discomfort in these areas.

Gentle neck and shoulder stretches can help relieve these problems and improve mobility.

### Day 1: Neck Tilt

- Sit comfortably on a chair with your feet flat on the floor.
- Breathe deeply while lengthening your spine.
- Exhale and gently tilt your head to the right, bringing your right ear toward your right shoulder.
- Hold the stretch for a few breaths, feeling a slight stretch along the left side of your neck.
- Inhale to return your head to a neutral position.
- Exhale and tilt your head to the left, bringing your left ear toward your left shoulder.
- Hold the stretch for a few breaths, feeling a slight stretch along the right side of your neck.
- Inhale to return your head to a neutral position.
- Repeat this sequence 5-10 times on each side.

Neck tilts are a great way to release tension in the neck and improve flexibility in this area.

## Day 2: Neck Rolls

Neck rolls can help relieve tension in the neck and improve circulation to the area.

- Sit comfortably on a chair with your feet flat on the floor.
- Breathe deeply while lengthening your spine.
- Exhale and gently lower your chin toward your chest.
- Inhale and slowly roll your head to the right, bringing your right ear toward your right shoulder.
- Exhale and continue to tilt your head back so that your chin points up.
- Inhale and roll your head to the left, bringing your left ear toward your left shoulder.
- Exhale and roll your head toward your chest.
- Repeat this circular motion, inhaling as you roll to the right and exhaling as you roll to the left.
- Continue for 5-10 cycles, then reverse the direction.

**NB:** Neck rolls should be slow and controlled to prevent any discomfort or strain.

This exercise can help to improve neck mobility and release tension.

## Day 3: Shoulder Rolls

Shoulder rolls are a simple but effective way to relieve tension in the shoulders and upper back.
- Sit comfortably on your chair with your feet flat on the floor.
- Inhale deeply, lengthening your spine.
- Exhale and lift your shoulders toward your ears.
- Inhale as you roll your shoulders back and down.
- Exhale as you roll your shoulders forward and up again.
- Repeat this shoulder roll movement for 1-2 minutes.

Shoulder rolls are a great way to release tension in the shoulders and improve circulation.
They are also helpful in promoting good posture.

## Day 4: Shoulder Blade Squeezes

Shoulder blade squeezes can help improve posture and alleviate discomfort in the upper back.

- Sit comfortably on your chair with your feet flat on the floor.
- Inhale deeply, lengthening your spine.
- Exhale and gently squeeze your shoulder blades together.
- Hold the squeeze for a few breaths.
- Inhale and release the pressure, letting your shoulders relax.
- Repeat this exercise for 1 to 2 minutes.

The shoulder press helps activate the muscles between the shoulder blades, which can become weak due to poor posture.


### Day 5: Combined  Neck and Shoulder Stretch

On day five, combine neck and shoulder stretch to completely relax your upper body.

- Sit comfortably on a chair with your feet flat on the floor.
- Breathe deeply while lengthening your spine.
- Exhale and tilt your head to the right, bringing your right ear toward your right shoulder.
- At the same time, lift your shoulders toward your ears.

- Hold this position for a few breaths.
- Inhale to return your head to a neutral position and lower your shoulders.
- Exhale and tilt your head to the left, bringing your left ear toward your left shoulder while lifting your shoulders.
- Hold this position for a few breaths.
- Inhale to return your head to a neutral position and lower your shoulders.
- Repeat this sequence 5 to 10 times on each side.

This combined stretch helps release tension in the neck and shoulders simultaneously, promoting relaxation and mobility in the upper body.

# 15-Minute Daily Routine

To wrap up our first week of chair yoga, we will develop a 15-minute daily routine that incorporates elements of breath awareness, relaxation, and light stretching gently on the neck and shoulders you have learned so far.

This routine is designed to be a gentle and effective way to start your daily chair yoga practice.

## Daily 15-Minute Routine

- Start by sitting comfortably on a chair with your feet flat on the floor and your hands resting on your knees.
- Close your eyes and take a few deep breaths to center yourself.
- Spend a few minutes practicing deep breathing, as you did on the first day, focusing on the rise and fall of your abdomen as you inhale and exhale.
- Move on to **guided relaxation (Day 2),** imagine your peaceful place, and allow yourself to relax completely for 5-10 minutes.
- Combine **breath and body awareness (Day 3)** to connect with different areas of your body, paying attention to areas of tension or discomfort.
- Move on to **stress-reducing breathing exercises (day 4),** using the 4-4-6 breathing pattern to activate the body's relaxation response for 5 to 10 minutes.
- Finish your routine by **combining your breathing with gentle movements (Day 5),** raising and lowering your arms in sync with your breathing for several minutes.
- Conclude your routine with the **combined neck and shoulder stretch (Day 5),** performing it on both sides to release tension and promote relaxation.

This 15-minute daily routine is an excellent way to start your chair yoga practice, as it provides a comprehensive approach to relaxation, stress reduction, and body awareness.

As you continue with your chair yoga journey in the weeks to come, you can gradually incorporate more physical exercises and stretches, building on the foundation you've established in Week 1.

# Chapter 2

## Week 2: Improving Flexibility with Chair Yoga for Seniors Over 60

Welcome to Week 2 of your Chair Yoga journey for seniors over 60. Building upon the foundational knowledge and skills you developed in Week 1, we now move our focus toward enhancing flexibility.

As we age, maintaining flexibility is vital for the health of our joints, muscles, and overall mobility.

Chair yoga offers a safe and effective way to work on flexibility, even for those with limited mobility or physical restrictions.

In this chapter, we'll explore a range of chair yoga poses and exercises designed to improve flexibility.

Whether you are new to yoga or have some experience, you will find these exercises beneficial for increasing your range of motion and promoting better joint health.

We'll also give you a daily 15-minute  routine all week to help you incorporate these flexibility-boosting exercises into your life.

# Days 6-12:  Chair Yoga Poses for Flexibility

Chair Yoga offers a  variety of positions that can be adapted to improve flexibility, making people over 60 years of age accessible.

Here, we'll introduce several poses that focus on different areas of the body and help enhance flexibility.

### Day 6: Seated Cat-Cow Stretch

The Seated Cat-Cow Stretch is a modified version of the traditional Cat-Cow pose, providing a gentle way to warm up and improve flexibility in the spine.

- Sit on your chair with your feet flat on the floor, hands resting on your knees.
- Inhale, arch your back, and lift your head, creating a gentle backbend (Cow).
- Exhale, round your back, and tuck your chin to your chest (Cat).
- Repeat this sequence inhaling into the cow and exhaling toward the cat for 1-2 minutes.

Seated crawl stretches are a great way to improve spinal flexibility, improve posture, and reduce back stiffness.

### Day 7: Seated Mountain Pose

Seated Mountain Pose helps improve posture and spinal flexibility.
- Sit with your feet flat on the floor and your hands on your knees.
- Inhale, lengthen your spine and straighten your arms overhead.
- Exhale, lower your arms and keep your spine tall.
- Repeat this movement, inhaling as you reach up and exhaling as you lower your arms for 1-2 minutes.

This pose stretches the spine and encourages proper alignment, which is essential for overall flexibility and posture.


**Day 8: Seated Forward Bend**

The Seated Forward Bend is excellent for stretching the hamstrings and lower back.

- Sit on your chair with your feet flat on the floor. Inhale, lengthen your spine.
- Exhale, hinge at your hips, and reach your hands towards your feet, rounding your back.
- Hold the stretch for 20-30 seconds, feeling a gentle stretch in your hamstrings and lower back.
- Inhale to return to an upright position.

This pose helps improve flexibility in the hamstrings and lower back, enhancing your ability to bend forward and reach your toes.

**Day 9: Seated Spinal Twist**

Seated Spinal Twist is an excellent position to improve spinal flexibility and promote better digestion.

- Sit on a chair with your feet flat on the floor.
- Inhale, lengthen your spine.
- Exhale, turn your body to the right, hold the back of the chair with your left hand, and place your right hand on the outside of your left thigh.
- Hold the twist for 20-30 seconds.
- Inhale to return to center.
- Exhale and repeat the twist on the other side.

Seated Spinal Twist improves spinal flexibility and promotes better digestion and elimination.

**Day 10: Seated Butterfly Pose**

Seated Butterfly Pose is great for improving flexibility in the hips and inner thighs.

- Sit on a chair with your feet flat on the floor.
- Inhale, lengthen your spine.
- Exhale, relax your knees to the sides, bringing the soles of your feet together.

- Use your hands to hold your legs and gently press your knees onto the floor.
- Hold the stretch for 20-30 seconds.
- Inhale to return your knees to an upright position.

This pose is a gentle way to improve hip and inner thigh flexibility, which can be particularly helpful for seniors.

**Day 11: Seated Pigeon Pose**

The Seated Pigeon Pose is a modified version of the traditional Pigeon pose, which focuses on hip flexibility.

- Sit on your chair with your feet flat on the floor.
- Inhale, lengthen your spine.
- Exhale, lift your right ankle and place it on your left thigh, flexing your right foot.
- Hold the stretch for 20-30 seconds.
- Inhale to bring your right leg back to the floor.
- Exhale and repeat the stretch with the left ankle resting on the right thigh.

Seated pigeon pose is a great way to improve hip flexibility and release tension in the hips.

Seated leg stretches are the perfect way to improve flexibility in the hamstrings and calves.

- Sit on  a chair with your feet flat on the floor.
- Inhale, lengthen your spine.
- Exhale, and stretch your right leg forward while bending it.
- Hold the stretch for 20-30 seconds.
- Inhale to bend your right knee and bring your foot back to the floor.
- Exhale, and repeat the stretch with your left leg.

This pose helps improve the flexibility of your hamstrings and calves, which can make everyday activities more comfortable.

# Seated Forward Bends and Twists

Seated forward bends and twists are essential components of chair yoga for improving flexibility.

They focus on stretching and mobilizing the spine, hamstrings, and hip area.


### Seated Forward Bend Sequence

The Seated Forward Bend Sequence combines several variations of the forward bend to stretch the spine, hamstrings, and lower back.

- Sit on a chair, feet flat on the floor, hands on knees.
- Inhale, lengthen your spine and raise your arms above your head.
- Exhale and bend your hips, reaching your arms toward your legs, and arching your back.
- Hold the stretch for 20-30 seconds.
- Inhale to return to an upright position.
- Exhale and repeat the forward bend, this time reaching one ankle, then the other.
- Inhale to return to an upright position.

This sequence helps improve spinal flexibility and stretches the hamstrings and lower back.


### Seated Spinal Twist Sequence

Seated Spinal Twist Sequence combines twists to improve spinal flexibility and release tension.

- Sit on a chair with your feet flat on the floor.
- Inhale, lengthen your spine.
 - Exhale and twist your torso to the right, holding the back of the chair with your left hand and placing your right hand on the outside of your left thigh.
- Hold the twist for 20-30 seconds.
- Inhale to return to the center.
- Exhale and repeat the twist on the other side.
- Inhale to return to the center.

This sequence enhances spinal flexibility and helps release tension in the spine.

# Leg Stretches

Leg stretches are essential for improving flexibility in the lower body, including the hamstrings, calves, and hip area.

### Leg Stretch Sequence

Leg Stretch Sequence incorporates several leg stretches to improve lower body flexibility.

- Sit on a chair, feet flat on the floor, hands on knees.
- Inhale, lengthen your spine.
- Exhale and stretch your right leg forward, flexing your foot.
- Hold the stretch for 20-30 seconds.
- Inhale to bend your right knee and return your foot to the floor.
- Exhale and repeat the stretch with the left leg.
- Inhale to bring your left leg back to the floor.
- Exhale, lift your right leg and place your right ankle on your left thigh.
- Hold the stretch for 20-30 seconds.
- Inhale to return your right foot to the floor.
- Exhale and repeat the stretch with your left leg on your right thigh.
- Inhale to return your left foot to the floor.

This sequence improves lower body flexibility by stretching the hamstrings, calves, and hips.

# 15 Minute Daily Routine

Now, let's create a 15-minute daily routine for week 2 that includes chair yoga poses, forward bends and twists, and leg stretches you have learned.

This routine is designed to help you gradually improve your flexibility and mobility.

## Daily 15-Minute Routine

- Start by sitting comfortably on a chair with your feet flat on the floor and your hands resting on your knees.

- Close your eyes and take a few deep breaths to center yourself.

- Spend a few minutes practicing deep breathing, as you did in Week 1, focusing on the rise and fall of your abdomen as you inhale and exhale.

- Moving on to **guided relaxation (day 2 of week 1),** imagine your peaceful place and allow yourself to relax completely for 5-10 minutes.

- Perform the **cat-cow stretch (day 6)** for 1-2 minutes, focusing on spinal flexibility.

- Perform the **seated forward bend (day 8)** for 20-30 seconds, gently stretching your hamstrings and lower back.

- Move into a **seated spinal twist (day 9)** for 20-30 seconds on each side to improve spinal flexibility.

- Perform the **Seated Mountain Pose (Day 7)** for 1-2 minutes, focusing on posture and spinal flexibility.

- Move into a **seated leg stretch(day 12)** for 20-30 seconds on each side to improve lower body flexibility.

- Finish your routine with the **seated butterfly pose (day 10)** for 20-30 seconds, improving hip and inner thigh flexibility.

- End your routine with a few deep breaths, inhaling, and exhaling to center yourself.

This 15-minute daily routine helps you gradually develop flexibility and mobility in different areas of your body, from your spine to your lower body and hips.

As you continue to practice these poses and stretches, you will notice increased flexibility and a greater sense of ease in your movements.

# Chapter 3

## Week 3: Enhancing Balance with Chair Yoga for Seniors Over 60

Welcome to the third week of your Chair Yoga journey for Seniors over 60.

In this chapter, we will focus on improving balance.

As we age, maintaining and improving balance becomes important to prevent falls and maintain independence.

Chair yoga offers a safe and effective way to maintain balance, even for people with limited mobility or physical limitations.

In this chapter, we will explore a series of chair yoga poses and exercises specifically designed to improve balance. Whether you're new to yoga or have some experience, you'll find these practices beneficial for improving your stability and coordination. We'll also provide you with a 15-minute daily routine for the entire week to help you integrate balance-enhancing exercises into your life.

# Days 13-19: Chair Yoga Poses for Balance

Chair yoga offers a variety of poses that can be adapted to improve balance and stability.
 Here, we'll introduce several poses that focus on different aspects of balance, from leg strength to overall stability.

### Day 13: Seated Leg Lifts
 Seated Leg Lifts are excellent for improving leg strength and balance.

- Sit on your chair with your feet flat on the floor, hands resting on your knees.
- Inhale, lengthen your spine.
- Exhale and lift your right leg straight out in front of you, engaging your core.
- Hold the leg lift for 20-30 seconds.
- Inhale to lower your right leg to the floor.
- Exhale and repeat the lift with your left leg.

- Inhale to lower your left leg to the floor.

This pose improves leg strength and challenges your balance and core stability.

### Day 14: Seated Warrior Pose

Seated Warrior Pose focuses on balance and stability while engaging the core.

- Sit on a chair with your feet flat on the floor.
- Inhale, lengthen your spine and raise your arms above your head.
- Exhale and twist your body to the right, holding the back of the chair with your left hand.
- Inhale to lift your right arm, keeping your spine straight.
- Hold the pose for 20-30 seconds.
- Exhale to return to the center.
- Inhale and rotate your body to the left, using your right hand to hold the back of the chair.
- Exhale and lift your left arm, keeping your spine straight.
- Hold the pose for 20-30 seconds.
- Inhale to return to center.

Seated Warrior Pose improves balance and core strength while also improving posture.

**Day 15: Seated Tree Pose**

Seated Tree Pose is a modified version of the traditional tree pose, focusing on balance and stability.

- Sit on a chair, feet flat on the floor, hands on knees.
- Inhale, lengthen your spine.
- Exhale and lift your right leg off the floor, placing it on your left calf or thigh.
- Hold the pose for 20-30 seconds.
- Inhale to lower your right leg to the floor.
- Exhale and repeat the pose with your left leg.

The seated Tree pose improves balance, stability, and leg strength.

**Day 16: Seated Eagle Pose**

Seated Eagle Pose targets balance and coordination.

- Sit on a chair, feet flat on the floor, hands on knees.
- Inhale, lengthen your spine.

- Exhale and cross your right thigh over your left
thigh, bringing your right foot behind your left calf.
- Cross your right arm over your left arm, bringing
your palms together.
- Hold the pose for 20-30 seconds.
 Inhale to relax your arms and legs.
- Exhale and repeat the pose with the left thigh
placed on the right thigh and the left arm placed on
the right arm.

 Seated Eagle Pose improves balance, coordination,
and concentration.


**Day 17: Seated Half Moon Pose**
 Seated Half Moon Pose improves balance and
stretches the sides of your body.

- Sit on a chair, feet flat on the floor, hands on
knees.
- Inhale, lengthen your spine.
- Exhale and bend to the right, bringing your right
hand toward the floor.
- Hold the pose for 20-30 seconds.
- Inhale to return to an upright position.
- Exhale and repeat the stretch to the left.

Seated Half Moon Pose improves balance, stretches the sides of your body, and enhances posture.


### Day 18: Seated Mountain Pose with Leg Lift

The Seated Mountain Pose with Leg Lift focuses on balance and leg strength.


- Sit on your chair with your feet flat on the floor, hands resting on your knees.
- Inhale, lengthen your spine and raise your arms above your head.
- Exhale and lift your right leg in front of you, tightening your body.
- Hold the leg lift for 20-30 seconds.
- Inhale to lower your right leg to the floor.
- Exhale and repeat the lift with your left leg.
- Inhale to lower your left leg to the floor.


This pose improves balance, leg strength, and overall stability.


### Day 19: Chair Pose

Chair Pose is a modified version of the traditional chair pose, focusing on balance and leg strength.

- Sit on a chair with your feet flat on the floor.
- Inhale, lengthen your spine.
- Exhale and raise your arms above your head, palms facing each other.
- Inhale to bend your knees and lower your hips toward the floor.
- Exhale and hold the sitting position in the chair for 20-30 seconds.

Chair Pose improves balance, leg strength, and core stability.

# Seated Side Stretches and Hip Openers

Seated Stretches and Hip Openers are essential for improving balance and stability because they target the hips, obliques, and inner thighs.

**Seated Side Stretch Sequence**

Seated Side Stretch Sequence combines stretches to improve balance and flexibility on both sides of your body.

- Sit on a chair, feet flat on the floor, hands on knees.
- Inhale, lengthen your spine.
- Exhale and bend to the right, bringing your right hand toward the floor.
- Hold the stretch for 20-30 seconds.
- Inhale to return to an upright position.
- Exhale and repeat the stretch to the left.

This sequence helps improve balance, stretches both sides of the body, and improves posture.

**Hip Opening Sequence**

The hip Opening Sequence incorporates stretches to open the hips, improve balance, and release tension in the hip area.

- Sit on a chair, feet flat on the floor, hands on knees.
- Inhale, lengthen your spine.
- Exhale and lift your right ankle and place it on your left thigh.

- Hold the stretch for 20-30 seconds.
- Inhale to bring your right leg back to the floor.
- Exhale and repeat the stretch with the left ankle resting on the right thigh.

   This sequence improves balance,  flexibility, and hip stability.

# Core-strengthening Exercises

A strong core is essential for balance and stability.
   In this section, we'll explore core strengthening exercises that can be incorporated into your chair yoga practice.

### Core Strengthening Sequence
   Core Strengthening Series combines exercises to improve core strength and stability.

- Sit on a chair, feet flat on the floor, hands on knees.
- Inhale, lengthen your spine.

- Exhale and contract your abdomen, drawing your navel toward your spine.
- Hold Core engagement for 20-30 seconds.
- Inhale to release and relax your body.
- Exhale and repeat the main movement.

This sequence strengthens the core muscles, enhancing balance and stability.

# 15-Minute Daily Routine

Now, let's put together a 15-minute daily routine for Week 3, which combines the chair yoga poses for balance, seated side stretches and hip openers, and core-strengthening exercises you've learned.

This routine is designed to help you gradually enhance your balance, stability, and coordination.

## 15-Minute Daily Routine

- Begin by sitting comfortably on your chair with your feet flat on the floor and your hands resting on your knees.

- Close your eyes and take a few deep breaths to center yourself.

- Spend a few minutes practicing deep breathing, as you have done in previous weeks, focusing on the rise and fall of your abdomen as you inhale and exhale.

- Moving on to **guided relaxation (day 2 of week 1),** imagine your peaceful place and allow yourself to relax completely for 5-10 minutes.

- Perform **seated leg lifts (day 13)** for 20-30 seconds on each leg to improve leg strength and balance.

- Move into **Seated Warrior Pose (day 14)** for 20-30 seconds on each side to improve balance and core strength.

- Perform **Seated Tree Pose (Day 15)** for 20-30 seconds on each leg to improve balance and stability.

- Perform **Seated Eagle Pose (Day 16)** for 20-30 seconds on each side to improve balance and coordination.

- Perform the **Seated Half Moon Pose (Day 17)** for 20-30 seconds on each side to improve balance and stretch both sides of the body.

- Move into **Seated mountain pose with leg lifts (day 18)** for 20-30 seconds on each leg to improve balance and leg strength.

- Do a **chair pose (day 19)** for 20-30 seconds to improve balance, leg strength, and core stability.

- Move into the **Seated Side Stretch Sequence**, stretching to the right and left for 20-30 seconds on each side to improve balance and flexibility in the sides of your body.

- Perform the **Hip Opener Sequence,** holding each stretch for 20-30 seconds, to improve balance and hip flexibility.

- Finish your routine with the **Core-Strengthening Sequence**, engaging and releasing your core for 1-2 minutes.

- Conclude your routine with a few deep breaths, inhaling, and exhaling to center yourself.

This 15-minute daily routine helps you gradually enhance your balance, stability, and coordination, while also strengthening your core.

As you continue to practice these exercises, you will notice improved stability and confidence in your movements.

# Chapter 4

## Week 4: Progressing to Intermediate and Advanced Levels with Chair Yoga for Seniors Over 60

Welcome to Week 4 of your Chair Yoga journey for seniors over 60. This week marks a significant milestone in your practice, as we'll delve into intermediate and advanced chair yoga poses and techniques.

By now, you've developed a solid foundation in chair yoga, including relaxation, flexibility, balance, and breath awareness.

Week 4 is designed to take your practice to the next level, challenging your body and mind while fostering continued physical and mental well-being.

In this chapter, we'll explore advanced chair yoga poses, how to combine them into flowing sequences, the practice of pranayama (breath control) for mindfulness, and a 15-minute daily routine that integrates these new elements.

By the end of this week, you'll have a better understanding of the potential of chair yoga to improve your overall health and quality of life.

# Days 20-30: Advanced Chair Yoga Poses

Week 4 features a selection of elevated chair yoga poses. These poses are designed to challenge your body, improve strength and flexibility, and improve your overall chair yoga practice.

While they are more physically demanding than the previous poses, they are still adapted for the chair and accessible for seniors over 60.

### Day 20: Seated Warrior III

Seated Warrior III is an advanced variation of the Seated Warrior Pose, focusing on balance and leg strength.

- Sit on your chair with your feet flat on the floor, hands resting on your knees.
- Inhale, lengthen your spine.
- Exhale and extend your right leg straight out in front of you, keeping it lifted.
- At the same time, lean your torso forward, creating a straight line from your fingertips to your right foot.
- Hold the pose for 20-30 seconds.
- Inhale to return to an upright position.
- Exhale and repeat the pose with the left leg.

Seated Warrior III improves balance, leg strength, and core stability.

**Day 21: Seated  Extended Triangle**
Seated  Extended Triangle is an advanced variation of the traditional Triangle pose, focusing on balance and spinal flexibility.

- Sit on a chair, feet flat on the floor, hands on knees.
- Inhale, lengthen your spine.
- Exhale and stretch your right leg forward, keeping it still.

- Place your left hand on the chair's seat and raise your right arm over your head, creating a straight line from your left arm to your right leg.
- Hold the pose for 20-30 seconds.
- Inhale to return to an upright position.
- Exhale and repeat the pose with the left leg.

  Seated Extended Triangle improves balance, spinal flexibility, and posture.

### Day 22: Seated Half Lotus

Seated Half Lotus is an advanced variation of the Seated Lotus pose, focusing on hip flexibility and balance.

- Sit on a chair, feet flat on the floor, hands on knees.
- Inhale, lengthen your spine.
- Exhale and lift your right leg, placing it on your left thigh.
- Hold the pose for 20-30 seconds.
- Inhale to bring your right leg back to the floor.
- Exhale and repeat the pose with your left leg resting on your right thigh.

  Seated Half Lotus improves flexibility, balance, and stretch of the inner thighs.

**Day 23: Seated Boat Pose**

Seated Boat Pose is an advanced variation of Boat Pose, focusing on core strength and balance.

- Sit on a chair, feet flat on the floor, hands on knees.
- Inhale, lengthen your spine.
- Exhale and lift both feet off the floor, bringing your shins parallel to the floor.
- Extend your arms forward, palms facing each other.
- Hold the pose for 20-30 seconds.
- Inhale to lower your legs to the floor.

Seated boat pose improves core strength and balance.


**Day 24: Seated Crow Pose**

Seated Crow Pose is an advanced variation of Crow Pose, focusing on arm and core strength and balance.

- Sit on a chair, feet flat on the floor, hands on knees.

- Inhale, lengthen your spine.
- Exhale and lean forward, placing your hands on the back of the chair.
- Lift your feet off the floor, bend your knees, and bring them toward your chest.
- Hold the pose for 20-30 seconds.
- Inhale to bring your feet back to the floor.

The seated crow pose challenges your arm and body strength as well as balance.

### Day 25: Seated Wheel Pose

Seated Wheel Pose is an advanced variation of wheel pose, focusing on back flexibility and balance.

- Sit on a chair, feet flat on the floor, hands on knees.
- Inhale, lengthen your spine.
- Exhale and lean back, placing your hands on the chair arms, fingers pointing toward your feet.
- Lift your hips and chest, creating a curve in your back.
- Hold the pose for 20 to 30 seconds.
- Inhale to return to an upright position.

Seated Wheel Pose improves back flexibility and balance.

# Combining Poses for a Flowing Sequence

In this section, we will learn how to combine the advanced chair yoga poses you have learned into a flowing sequence.

Flowing sequences help you improve flexibility, strength, and coordination while promoting mindfulness and relaxation.

### Flowing Sequence 1

Flow Sequence 1 combines Seated Warrior III, Seated Half Lotus Pose, and Seated Boat Pose to create a dynamic flow.

- Start by sitting comfortably in a chair with your feet flat on the floor and your hands on your knees.
- Inhale, lengthen your spine.

- Exhale and stretch your right leg into Seated Warrior III, leaning your torso forward.
- Inhale and return to an upright position.
- Exhale and bring your right leg into the cross-legged position.
- Inhale and release your right leg to the floor.
- Exhale and lift both legs into a seated boat position, reaching your arms forward.
- Inhale to lower your legs to the floor.
- Repeat the sequence on the left side, starting with Seated Warrior III.

Flowing Sequence 1 improves balance, hip flexibility, core strength, and coordination.


**Flowing Sequence 2**

Flowing Sequence 2 combines the seated extended triangle, seated crow pose, and seated wheel pose to create a dynamic flow.

- Start by sitting comfortably on a chair with your feet flat on the floor and your hands on your knees.
- Inhale, lengthen your spine.
- Exhale and stretch your right leg into a seated kard.
- Inhale and return to an upright position.

- Exhale and lean back into the wheel position, creating a curve in your back.
- Inhale to return to an upright position.
- Repeat the sequence on the left side, starting with the seated extended triangle.

Flowing Sequence 2 improves balance, arm and core strength, flexibility, and back coordination.

# Pranayama Techniques for Mindfulness

Pranayama, or controlled breathing technique, is a fundamental aspect of yoga practice that can significantly improve your mindfulness, reduce stress, and promote relaxation.

In week 4, we'll explore two pranayama techniques to incorporate into your chair yoga practice.

Pranayama Technique 1: Bhramari (Bee Breath)

Bhramari, or Bee Breath, is a calming pranayama technique that helps reduce stress and anxiety while promoting a sense of inner peace.

- Sit comfortably on a chair and close your eyes.
- Take a deep breath through your nose.
- Exhale slowly, making a buzzing sound like a bee, cover your ears with your thumbs and gently press your fingers into your eyes.
- Repeat this humming sound for 3-5 breathing cycles.

 Bhramari is a great technique to relax and cultivate mindfulness during your chair yoga practice.


Pranayama Technique 2: Nadi Shodhana (Alternate Nostril Breathing)

Nadi Shodhana, or Alternate Nostril Breathing, is a balancing pranayama technique that harmonizes the body and mind.

- Sit comfortably on a chair and close your eyes.

- Place the right thumb on the right nostril and the right ring finger on the left nostril.
- Inhale deeply through the left nostril.
- Close the left nostril with the ring finger and exhale through the right nostril.
- Inhale through the right nostril.
- Close your right nostril with your thumb and exhale through your left nostril.
- Repeat this cycle for 3-5 minutes.

  Nadi Shodhana promotes mental clarity, balance, and mindfulness.


# 15-Minute Daily Routine

Now, let's create a 15-minute daily routine for Week 4, incorporating advanced chair yoga poses, flowing sequences, and pranayama techniques.

This routine is designed to challenge you physically and mentally while fostering relaxation and mindfulness.

# 15-Minute Daily Routine

- Begin by sitting comfortably on your chair with your feet flat on the floor and your hands resting on your knees.

- Close your eyes and take a few deep breaths to center yourself.

- Spend a few minutes practicing deep breathing, as you did in the previous weeks, focusing on the rise and fall of your abdomen as you breathe in and out.

- Transition into **guided relaxation (Day 2 of Week 1),** imagining your peaceful place and allowing yourself to fully relax for 5-10 minutes.

- Perform **Seated Warrior III (Day 20)** for 20-30 seconds on each leg to enhance balance, leg strength, and core stability.

- Move into **Flowing Sequence 1**, combining **Seated Warrior III, Seated Half Lotus, and Seated Boat Pose.**

- Transition into **Seated Extended Triangle (Day 21)** for 20-30 seconds on each side to improve balance, spinal flexibility, and posture.

- Move into **Flowing Sequence 2,** combining **Seated Extended Triangle, Seated Crow Pose, and Seated Wheel Pose.**

- Practice **Bhramari (Bee Breath)** for 3-5 breath cycles to promote relaxation and mindfulness.

- Perform **Seated Half Lotus (Day 22)** for 20-30 seconds on each leg to improve hip flexibility, balance, and inner thigh stretch.

- Move into **Seated Crow Pose (Day 23)** for 20-30 seconds to challenge arm and core strength, as well as balance.

- Practice **Nadi Shodhana (Alternate Nostril Breathing)** for 3-5 minutes to enhance mental clarity and balance.

- Perform **Seated Wheel Pose (Day 24)** for 20-30 seconds to improve back flexibility and balance.

- Finish your routine with a few deep breaths, inhaling, and exhaling to center yourself.

This 15-minute daily routine challenges you physically and mentally, while promoting relaxation, mindfulness, and a deeper understanding of the potential of chair yoga for your overall well-being.

# Chapter 5

## Meal Plans for Seniors Practicing Chair Yoga

In your journey of chair yoga for seniors over 60, you have learned the importance of staying active Be active and attentive through yoga practice.

However, good nutrition is an equally essential part of maintaining your overall health.

A balanced diet not only promotes physical health but also contributes to mental and emotional health.

It complements your chair yoga practice by providing the energy and nutrients your body needs.

This chapter is dedicated to developing a comprehensive meal plan specifically designed for seniors practicing chair yoga.

It includes information on a balanced diet, a 30-day meal plan with breakfast options, lunch and dinner ideas, snack options, and hydration tips. Additionally, we will cover special dietary considerations for older adults, ensuring that you know how to maintain a nutritious diet that complements your chair yoga practice.

# Balanced Nutrition for Seniors

Before diving into the 30-day meal plan, it is essential to understand what balanced nutrition for seniors means.

As you age, your nutritional needs change and it is important to adjust your diet accordingly.

Here are some key principles for seniors nutrition:

## 1. Calorie needs

Seniors generally need fewer calories than younger people because metabolism naturally slows with age. However, maintaining a balanced calorie intake is essential to support energy levels and overall health.

Consult a healthcare professional to determine your specific calorie needs.

## 2. Protein

Protein is essential for maintaining muscle mass, bone health, and overall physical function.

Try to include lean sources of protein in your diet, such as poultry, fish, beans, and dairy products.

For vegetarians, legumes, tofu, and dairy products can be excellent sources of protein.

## 3. Fiber

Fiber supports digestive health and helps control weight and blood sugar levels.

Incorporate fiber-rich foods like whole grains, fruits, vegetables, and legumes into your diet.

## 4. Vitamins and minerals

Older adults need specific vitamins and minerals, such as calcium and vitamin D for bone health and vitamin B12 for nerve function.

Make sure your diet includes a variety of nutrient-rich foods and consider taking a supplement if recommended by your healthcare professional.

## 5. Hydration

Dehydration is a common concern for older adults. Make it a habit to drink plenty of water throughout the day and include hydrating foods like fruits and vegetables in your meals.

## 6. Variety

A diverse diet helps you get a variety of nutrients.
 Explore different foods and flavors to keep your meals interesting and nutritious.

## 7. Portion Control

Pay attention to portion sizes to avoid overeating.
 Smaller, more frequent meals can help control calorie intake and support digestion.
 Now that you understand the principles of balanced nutrition for seniors, let's move on to the 30-day meal plan.

# 30-Day Meal Plan

## Week 1

**Day 1:**

**Breakfast:** Scrambled eggs with spinach and whole-grain toast.

**Lunch:** Grilled chicken salad with mixed greens, cherry tomatoes, and balsamic vinaigrette.

**Dinner:** Baked salmon with quinoa and steamed broccoli.

**Snack:** Greek yogurt with honey and a handful of almonds.

**Hydration:** Drink water, herbal tea, or water infused with lemon or cucumber throughout the day.

**Day 2:**

**Breakfast:** Oatmeal with sliced bananas, chopped nuts, and a drizzle of honey.

**Lunch:** Lentil soup with a side of whole-grain bread.

**Dinner:** Roasted turkey breast with sweet potato and sautéed green beans.

**Snack:** Carrot and celery sticks with hummus.

**Hydration:** Stay hydrated with water and herbal tea.

Day 3:

**Breakfast:** Whole-grain cereal with low-fat milk and fresh berries.

**Lunch:** Quinoa salad with chickpeas, cucumber, and feta cheese.

**Dinner:** Stir-fried tofu with brown rice and mixed vegetables.

**Snack:** A small apple with a tablespoon of almond butter.

**Hydration:** Consume water and herbal tea throughout the day.

**Breakfast:** Cottage cheese with sliced peaches and a sprinkle of cinnamon.

**Lunch:** Spinach and mushroom frittata with a side of mixed greens.

**Dinner:** Baked cod with wild rice and roasted Brussels sprouts.

**Snack:** A handful of walnuts and dried apricots.

**Hydration:** Keep up with water and herbal tea intake.

Day 5:

**Breakfast:** Whole-grain waffles with a dollop of Greek yogurt and fresh strawberries.

**Lunch:** Tomato and basil soup with a whole-grain roll.

**Dinner:** Grilled shrimp with quinoa and steamed asparagus.

**Snack:** Sliced cucumber with a light ranch dressing.

**Hydration:** Stay hydrated with water and herbal tea.

Day 6:

**Breakfast:** Scrambled tofu with diced bell peppers and a whole-grain English muffin.

**Lunch:** Chickpea and vegetable stew with a side of whole-grain crackers.

**Dinner:** Grilled chicken breast with brown rice and sautéed zucchini.

**Snack:** A small bunch of grapes.

**Hydration:** Continue to drink water and herbal tea.

Day 7:

**Breakfast:** Smoothie with low-fat yogurt, banana, spinach, and a scoop of protein powder.

**Lunch:** Quinoa salad with mixed vegetables and a tahini dressing.

**Dinner:** Baked trout with quinoa and roasted carrots.

**Snack:** Sliced bell peppers with guacamole.

**Hydration:** Maintain your water and herbal tea intake.

## Week 2

**Day 8:**

**Breakfast:** Whole-grain pancakes with fresh blueberries and a drizzle of maple syrup.

**Lunch:** Lentil and vegetable stir-fry with brown rice.

**Dinner:** Baked chicken with mashed sweet potatoes and steamed broccoli.

**Snack:** A handful of mixed nuts.

**Hydration:** Drink water and herbal tea throughout the day.



**Breakfast:** Greek yogurt parfait with granola and mixed berries.

**Lunch:** Spinach and feta stuffed chicken breast with a side of quinoa.

**Dinner:** Baked cod with brown rice and sautéed asparagus.

**Snack:** Sliced cucumber with tzatziki sauce.

**Hydration:** Stay hydrated with water and herbal tea.



**Breakfast:** Scrambled eggs with diced tomatoes and whole-grain toast.

**Lunch:** Minestrone with a side of whole-grain bread.

**Dinner:** Grilled shrimp with quinoa and roasted Brussels sprouts.

**Snack:** A small apple with a tablespoon of almond butter.

**Hydration:** Continue to drink water and herbal tea.


**Day 11:**

**Breakfast:** Oatmeal with sliced bananas, chopped nuts, and a drizzle of honey.

**Lunch:** Grilled chicken salad with mixed greens, cherry tomatoes, and balsamic vinaigrette.

**Dinner:** Stir-fried tofu with brown rice and mixed vegetables.

**Snack:** A handful of walnuts and dried apricots.

**Hydration:** Keep up with water and herbal tea intake.


**Day 12:**

**Breakfast:** Whole-grain cereal with low-fat milk and fresh berries.

**Lunch:** Tomato and basil soup with a whole-grain roll.

**Dinner:** Roasted turkey breast with sweet potato and sautéed green beans.

**Snack:** Sliced bell peppers with hummus.

**Hydration:** Stay hydrated with water and herbal tea.

Day 13:

**Breakfast:** Cottage cheese with sliced peaches and a sprinkle of cinnamon.

**Lunch:** Quinoa salad with chickpeas, cucumber, and feta cheese.

**Dinner:** Baked salmon with quinoa and steamed broccoli.

**Snack:** A small bunch of grapes.

**Hydration:** Continue to drink water and herbal tea.

**Day 14:**

**Breakfast:** Scrambled tofu with diced bell peppers and a whole-grain English muffin.

**Lunch:** Chickpea and vegetable stew with a side of whole-grain crackers.

**Dinner:** Baked trout with quinoa and roasted carrots.

**Snack:** Sliced cucumber with tzatziki sauce.

**Hydration:** Maintain your water and herbal tea intake.

## Week 3

**Day 15:**

**Breakfast:** Whole-grain waffles with a dollop of Greek yogurt and fresh strawberries.

**Lunch:** Spinach and mushroom frittata with a side of mixed greens.

**Dinner:** Baked chicken breast with brown rice and sautéed zucchini.

**Snack:** Greek yogurt with honey and a handful of almonds.

**Hydration:** Drink water and herbal tea throughout the day.

## Day 16:

**Breakfast:** Smoothie with low-fat yogurt, banana, spinach, and a scoop of protein powder.

**Lunch:** Quinoa salad with mixed vegetables and a tahini dressing.

**Dinner:** Grilled chicken breast with quinoa and steamed asparagus.

**Snack:** Carrot and celery sticks with hummus.

**Hydration:** Stay hydrated with water and herbal tea.

**Day 17:**

**Breakfast:** Scrambled eggs with spinach and whole-grain toast.

**Lunch:** Lentil and vegetable stir-fry with brown rice.

**Dinner:** Baked salmon with quinoa and roasted Brussels sprouts.

**Snack:** A handful of mixed nuts.

**Hydration:** Continue to drink water and herbal tea.

**Day 18:**

**Breakfast:** Greek yogurt parfait with granola and mixed berries.

**Lunch:** Quinoa salad with chickpeas, cucumber, and feta cheese.

**Dinner:** Grilled shrimp with quinoa and roasted carrots.

**Snack:** Sliced cucumber with a light ranch dressing.

**Hydration:** Keep up with water and herbal tea intake.

**Day 19:**

**Breakfast:** Whole-grain pancakes with fresh blueberries and a drizzle of maple syrup.

**Lunch:** Lentil soup with a side of whole-grain bread.

**Dinner:** Baked cod with brown rice and sautéed asparagus.

**Snack:** Sliced cucumber with tzatziki sauce.

**Hydration:** Stay hydrated with water and herbal tea.

**Day 20:**

**Breakfast:** Oatmeal with sliced bananas, chopped nuts, and a drizzle of honey.

**Lunch:** Spinach and feta stuffed chicken breast with a side of quinoa.

**Dinner:** Grilled shrimp with quinoa and roasted Brussels sprouts.

**Snack:** A small apple with a tablespoon of almond butter.

**Hydration:** Continue to drink water and herbal tea.

## Week 4

**Day 21:**

**Breakfast:** Whole-grain cereal with low-fat milk and fresh berries.

**Lunch:** Grilled chicken salad with mixed greens, cherry tomatoes, and balsamic vinaigrette.

**Dinner:** Stir-fried tofu with brown rice and mixed vegetables.

**Snack:** A handful of walnuts and dried apricots.

**Hydration:** Keep up with water and herbal tea intake.

**Day 22:**

**Breakfast:** Cottage cheese with sliced peaches and a sprinkle of cinnamon.

**Lunch:** Tomato and basil soup with a whole-grain roll.

**Dinner:** Roasted turkey breast with sweet potato and sautéed green beans.

**Snack:** Sliced bell peppers with hummus.

**Hydration:** Stay hydrated with water and herbal tea.

**Day 23:**

**Breakfast:** Scrambled tofu with diced bell peppers and a whole-grain English muffin.

**Lunch:** Chickpea and vegetable stew with a side of whole-grain crackers.

**Dinner:** Baked cod with wild rice and roasted Brussels sprouts.

**Snack:** A small bunch of grapes.

**Hydration:** Continue to drink water and herbal tea.


**Day 24:**

**Breakfast:** Whole-grain waffles with a dollop of Greek yogurt and fresh strawberries.

**Lunch:** Quinoa salad with mixed vegetables and a tahini dressing.

**Dinner:** Baked chicken with mashed sweet potatoes and steamed broccoli.

**Snack:** Sliced cucumber with a light ranch dressing.

**Hydration:** Keep up with water and herbal tea intake.


**Day 25:**

**Breakfast:** Smoothie with low-fat yogurt, banana, spinach, and a scoop of protein powder.

**Lunch:** Quinoa salad with chickpeas, cucumber, and feta cheese.

**Dinner:** Grilled chicken breast with brown rice and sautéed zucchini.

**Snack:** A small apple with a tablespoon of almond butter.

**Hydration:** Stay hydrated with water and herbal tea.


**Day 26:**

**Breakfast:** Scrambled eggs with diced tomatoes and whole-grain toast.

**Lunch:** Minestrone soup with a side of whole-grain bread.

**Dinner:** Baked salmon with quinoa and steamed broccoli.

**Snack:** Sliced cucumber with tzatziki sauce.

**Hydration:** Continue to drink water and herbal tea.

Day 27:

**Breakfast:** Greek yogurt parfait with granola and mixed berries.

**Lunch:** Lentil and vegetable stir-fry with brown rice.

**Dinner:** Baked trout with quinoa and roasted carrots.

**Snack:** A handful of mixed nuts.

**Hydration:** Stay hydrated with water and herbal tea.

Day 28:

**Breakfast:** Oatmeal with sliced bananas, chopped nuts, and a drizzle of honey.

**Lunch:** Spinach and feta stuffed chicken breast with a side of quinoa.

**Dinner:** Grilled shrimp with quinoa and roasted Brussels sprouts.

**Snack:** Sliced cucumber with a light ranch dressing.

**Hydration:** Keep up with water and herbal tea intake.

**Day 29:**

**Breakfast:** Whole-grain pancakes with fresh blueberries and a drizzle of maple syrup.

**Lunch:** Lentil soup with a side of whole-grain bread.

**Dinner:** Baked cod with brown rice and sautéed asparagus.

**Snack:** A small apple with a tablespoon of almond butter.

**Hydration:** Continue to drink water and herbal tea.

Day 30:

**Breakfast:** Smoothie with low-fat yogurt, banana, spinach, and a scoop of protein powder.

**Lunch:** Quinoa salad with mixed vegetables and a tahini dressing.

**Dinner:** Grilled chicken breast with quinoa and steamed asparagus.

**Snack:** Carrot and celery sticks with hummus.

**Hydration:** Stay hydrated with water and herbal tea

# Snacks and Hydration Tips

Snacks can be an essential part of your daily diet. It forms a source of energy between meals and helps maintain your metabolism.

Here are some healthy snack ideas suitable for seniors doing chair yoga:

**Nuts:** A small handful of mixed nuts (almonds, walnuts, or cashews) can make a satisfying and nutritious snack.

**Greek Yogurt:** A cup of Greek yogurt with a little honey and some fresh berries provides protein and probiotics.

**Sliced vegetables:** Carrots and celery or cucumber slices with hummus are a refreshing and healthy snack.

**Fresh Fruit:** Apples, grapes, and small bananas are convenient and portable options.

**Dried Fruit:** A handful of dried apricots, raisins, or figs can satisfy your sweet tooth.

**Nut Butter:** A tablespoon of almond or peanut butter pairs well with apple slices or whole-grain crackers.

**Cottage Cheese:** A serving of low-fat cottage cheese with sliced peaches or pineapple can be a tasty and protein-rich snack.

**Smoothies:** Blend low-fat yogurt, fruits, and a scoop of protein powder for a nutritious and hydrating snack.

Remember to stay well-hydrated throughout the day.

Proper hydration is crucial for overall health, and it complements your chair yoga practice by ensuring that your body can function optimally.

Here are some hydration tips for seniors:

**Water:** Drinking plain water is the best way to stay hydrated.

Aim to consume at least 8-10 cups of water per day, but your individual needs may vary.

**Herbal Tea:** Herbal teas, such as chamomile or peppermint, can be a soothing and hydrating choice.

**Water-Infused with Flavor:** If plain water feels dull, infuse it with slices of lemon, cucumber, or berries for a refreshing taste.

**Coconut Water:** Coconut water is a natural source of electrolytes and can be a good choice for rehydration.

**Low-Sugar Fruit Juices:** Occasionally, you can enjoy small servings of 100% fruit juices, but be mindful of their sugar content.

**Milk or Milk Alternatives:** Low-fat milk or dairy alternatives like almond or soy milk can contribute to your daily fluid intake.

# Special Dietary Considerations for Seniors

As a senior, you may have specific dietary considerations or restrictions based on your health and medical conditions.

It is essential to consult with a healthcare professional or registered dietitian to address these concerns.

Here are some common dietary considerations for older adults:

**1. Sodium intake:** Many older adults need to monitor their sodium intake, especially if they have blood pressure High.

Reducing salt in your diet can help reduce your risk of cardiovascular problems.

Choose low-sodium or salt-free options when available.

**2. Fiber:** Adequate fiber intake is essential for digestive health, but some older adults may need to be careful with high-fiber foods, especially if they have sugar problems Digest.

In such cases, consult a healthcare professional to find the appropriate balance.

**3. Calcium and vitamin D:** Older people often need more calcium and vitamin D to maintain bone health.

Include dairy products, leafy greens, and fortified foods in your diet, and consider supplements if recommended.

**4. Special Diets:** If you have specific dietary needs, such as a vegetarian or vegan diet, diabetic diet, or gluten-free diet, work with a dietitian to ensure you're meeting your nutritional requirements while adhering to your dietary preferences or restrictions.

**5. Food Allergies:** Be aware of food allergies or sensitivities, and avoid foods that trigger adverse reactions.

For those with food allergies, it's important to read food labels carefully.

**6. Medication Interactions:** Some foods or beverages may interact with medications.

Consult with your healthcare provider to ensure your diet doesn't interfere with your prescribed medications.

**7. Digestive problems:** Older adults may experience digestive changes, such as constipation or gastrointestinal discomfort.

Increasing fiber intake, drinking plenty of water, and eating foods rich in probiotics can help alleviate these problems.

# Chapter 6

# Practical Tips for Seniors Practicing Chair Yoga

As a senior starting your chair yoga journey, you have taken a positive step in improving your physical health substance, and spirit.

Chair yoga offers many benefits, including improved flexibility, balance, strength, and relaxation.

It's a safe and accessible way to stay active and maintain your health as you age.

This chapter is dedicated to giving you practical tips for getting the most out of your chair yoga practice. We'll cover safety precautions and contraindications, how to use props and modifications, and establish a comfortable and motivating practice space while tracking your progress.

This information will help you create a fulfilling and sustainable chair yoga routine to improve your overall quality of life.

# Safety Precautions and Contraindications

Before beginning chair yoga, it is essential to understand safety precautions and be aware of any contraindications.

Safety should always be a top priority as it ensures that your operations are not only efficient but also risk-free.

## Safety Precautions

**Consult your healthcare provider:** If you have any health conditions, especially if they are chronic or require treatment continuously, consult your healthcare provider before starting chair yoga.

They can tell you whether chair yoga is right for you and whether any modifications are needed.

**Start slowly:** If you're new to chair yoga or haven't been active in a while, start slowly and gradually increase the duration and intensity of your workout. This gradual approach minimizes the risk of strain or injury.

**Stay hydrated:** Proper hydration is important for maintaining overall health. Drink water before, during, and after chair yoga to avoid dehydration.

**Use the right chair:** Make sure the chair you use is stable and has a backrest. Avoid using chairs with wheels as they may not provide the necessary stability. Also, check the chair for any sharp edges or parts that could cause discomfort during exercise.

**Wear comfortable clothes:** Choose loose, breathable clothes that help you move easily. Avoid wearing clothes with belts or accessories that can dig into your skin when you are in a sitting or reclining position.

**Practice in a Well-Lit Space:** Ensure your practice space is well-lit to prevent accidents and make it easier to follow instructions.

**Listen to Your Body:** Pay close attention to your body's signals.

If you experience pain, discomfort, or dizziness during any pose, stop immediately and consult with a healthcare professional if necessary.

## Contraindications

Although chair yoga is generally safe for older adults, certain medical conditions or conditions may contraindicate certain positions or practices.
Note the following contraindications:

**Recent surgery:** If you have recently had surgery, consult your surgeon or healthcare professional before practicing chair yoga.
Some post-operative restrictions may apply.

**Severe joint pain:** If you have severe joint pain, avoid positions that make the pain worse.
Gentle movements are usually recommended but talk to your doctor for advice.

**Uncontrolled high blood pressure:** If your blood pressure is uncontrolled or excessively high, consult your health care professional before starting chair yoga.

**Dizziness or vertigo:** If you have a history of dizziness or experience frequent dizziness, avoid positions that involve rapid or excessive head movements.

**Glaucoma:** Certain yoga poses that involve inverting the head may increase intraocular pressure and are contraindicated for people with glaucoma.

**Recent fracture or injury:** If you have recently suffered a fracture or injury, consult a health care professional or physical therapist to determine if chair yoga is suitable for you.

**Pregnancy:** If you are pregnant, consult your health care professional before practicing chair yoga.
  Certain positions and practices may need to be modified or avoided.

# Using Props and Modifications

Chair Yoga can be adjusted to meet your individual needs and abilities through the use of props and modifications.

Props can enhance your workout by providing support, stability, and comfort.

## Common Props for Chair Yoga

**Chair:** Your main accessory is of course the chair. Choose a sturdy, stable chair with a backrest.

**Yoga Strap:** Yoga Strap can be used for stretching and reaching exercises, giving you access to a wider range of motion.

**Yoga Blocks:** Yoga blocks can be placed under your feet or hands to assist with balance and alignment in certain poses.

**Cushions or pillows:** Placing cushions or pillows on the seat of your chair can make sitting more comfortable and reduce pressure on your hips and lower back.

**Blanket:** A folded blanket can add support to sitting positions and make relaxing positions more comfortable.

## Modifications

Chair yoga can be adjusted to accommodate different physical abilities and limitations.
Here are some common modifications to consider:

**Reduced range of motion:** If your range of motion is limited, focus on smaller movements.
For example, if you can't raise your arms above your head, simply raise them to a comfortable height.

**Lower Intensity:** If you're looking for a low-intensity workout, choose gentler positions and movements.
Gradually progress to more difficult poses as your strength and flexibility improve.

**Balance support:** For poses that challenge your balance, keep a chair nearby to hold on if needed.
You can also bring your feet closer together to increase stability.

**Seated Variations:** If standing poses are difficult, look for seated variations of these poses.
For example, Seated Mountain Pose is the seated version of the traditional Mountain Pose.

**Use props:** Don't hesitate to use accessories such as cushions or pillows to feel more comfortable when sitting or relaxing.

**Supported positions:** For relaxation positions, use props such as folded blankets under the head and neck to provide comfort and relaxation.

**Breathing Techniques:** Incorporate gentle breathing and relaxation techniques to enhance your exercise and reduce stress.

**Adaptive seating:** Some people who practice chair yoga may use a wheelchair or mobility aid.
In such cases, the chair yoga can still be adjusted to your needs.

Focus on sitting positions and movements that you can do comfortably in a chair.
Remember that chair yoga is highly customizable and it's important to practice it in a way that is safe and comfortable for you.

Feel free to experiment with different accessories and modifications to find what works best for your unique body and needs.

# Setting up a Comfortable Practice Space

Creating a comfortable practice space is essential to enjoying your chair yoga sessions. A friendly environment can make your workouts more enjoyable and keep you motivated.

Here are some tips for setting up a comfortable practice space:

### 1. Choose a Quiet Space

Find a quiet, peaceful space where you can practice without distractions.

If possible, let your family or roommates know when you'll be exercising so they don't bother you.

## 2. Gather Your Equipment

Gather all the props and equipment you need for your chair yoga session.

Having everything ready before you begin will help you stay focused and avoid interruptions.

## 3. Adequate lighting

Make sure the room is well-lit.

Good lighting is important for safety and following instructions during your workout.

## 4. Comfortable Chair

Use a comfortable and stable chair with a backrest.

It should have the right height and width to support your body during exercise.

## 5. Supportive Flooring

If you are doing the standing pose, make sure the floor is supportive and not too slippery.

A non-slip yoga mat can be placed under your chair if necessary.

## 6. Personalize your space

Add personal touches to your workout space, like calming artwork, soft colors, or even potted plants.

This can create a calming and pleasant atmosphere.


### 7. Music or Soundscapes

Some people find that soothing background music or nature sounds enhance their exercise.

Experiment with different sounds to see which sounds most relaxing to you.


### 8. Temperature Control

Maintain a comfortable temperature in your practice space. You don't want to be too hot or too cold, as this can be distracting.


### 9. Stay Organized

Keep your practice space organized.

Arrange your props neatly so that you can access them easily. Clutter can be distracting.


### 10. Make It Personal

Consider adding a small personal altar or a space for meditation if you're interested in including these aspects in your practice.

Remember, your practice space should be a place of comfort and peace.

Tailor it to your preferences and make it a space where you look forward to practicing chair yoga.

# Staying Motivated and Tracking Progress

Maintaining motivation and tracking your progress is essential for a fulfilling chair yoga practice.

Here are some tips to help you stay motivated and monitor your improvement:

### 1. Set Clear Goals

Establish specific, realistic goals for your chair yoga practice. Your goals can be related to flexibility, balance, strength, or stress reduction.

Having clear goals gives you meaning and direction.

## 2. Create a habit

Consistency is the key to progress. Establish a regular chair yoga routine, whether daily, several times a week, or every other week.

Set aside time specifically for your practice and make it a non-negotiable part of your schedule.

## 3. Use a journal

Keep a chair yoga journal to record your experiences, goals, and progress. Record how you feel before and after each workout session and note any changes in your physical or mental health.

A journal can also be a source of motivation as you see how far you have come.

## 4. Find a Practice Partner

If you enjoy social interactions, consider practicing chair yoga with a friend or family member.

You can motivate each other, share experiences, and make it a fun and social activity.

## 5. Online Communities

Join online chair yoga communities or forums where you can connect with like-minded individuals.

Sharing your journey and experiences with others can be motivating, and you can learn from others as well.

## 6. Celebrate your achievements

Celebrate your achievements, no matter how small they may seem. Realizing your progress can be very motivating.

Treat yourself to something special or reward yourself when you reach a goal.

## 7. Stay Informed

Continue learning about chair yoga by reading books, watching videos, or taking online classes.

Gaining knowledge of the practice can help you maintain interest.

## 8. Ask for advice

If you feel stuck or need advice, consider working with a chair yoga instructor or joining group classes.

Instructors can provide personalized feedback and guidance to help you improve.

## 9. Visualize success

Visualize yourself successfully completing difficult poses and achieving your goals.
 Visualization can be a powerful motivator and can increase confidence in your abilities.

## 10. Embrace mindfulness

Incorporate mindfulness practices into your chair yoga routine. Mindfulness can help you stay present in the moment, reduce stress, and maintain a positive attitude toward your practice.

## 11. Track Physical Changes

 Record the physical changes you notice as you progress through your chair yoga practice.
 Can you go further at once?
 Has your balance improved?
 Do you feel stronger?
 These tangible improvements can be very motivating.

## 12. Adapt and modify

As you gain experience with chair yoga, adapt and modify your practice to keep it interesting and challenging.

Explore new poses and variations to avoid boredom and stagnation.

Staying motivated and tracking progress with your chair yoga practice is an ongoing process.

It requires dedication, self-compassion, and the willingness to embrace the journey as much as the destination.

Remember that chair yoga is a practice, and with patience and persistence, you'll experience the numerous physical and mental benefits it offers.

# Conclusion

As we conclude our exploration of chair yoga for seniors over 60, it's essential to reflect on the long-term benefits of this practice, encourage its continuation beyond the initial 30 days, and provide additional resources for further exploration.

Chair yoga is not just a temporary fitness regimen; it's a path to improved physical health, mental well-being, and an overall enhanced quality of life.

Let's delve into these important aspects.

## The Long-Term Benefits of Chair Yoga for Seniors

Chair yoga offers a multitude of long-term benefits that can positively impact the lives of seniors.

Its gentle, accessible nature makes it an ideal practice for those seeking to maintain and improve their well-being in the later stages of life.

Here are some of the enduring advantages of chair yoga:

## 1. Enhanced Flexibility

Regular chair yoga practice gradually increases your flexibility. This is especially significant for seniors, as improved flexibility can ease the discomfort of stiff joints and muscles, enhance mobility, and make daily activities more manageable.

## 2. Improve balance

One of the main concerns of older adults is the risk of falls. Chair yoga combines postures and balance-enhancing exercises that can significantly reduce the risk of falls and injuries.

## 3. Strength Building

Over time, chair yoga helps strengthen muscles and improve functional strength. This makes daily tasks easier, leading to a more active and independent lifestyle.

## 4. Pain Management

Older adults often struggle with various forms of chronic pain, such as arthritis or lower back pain. Chair yoga reduces this discomfort and may reduce the need for pain medication.

## 5. Mental Clarity and Stress Reduction

The relaxation and mindfulness components of chair yoga help improve mental clarity and reduce stress. These aspects are invaluable for older adults who want to maintain their cognitive and mental health.

## 6. Better Posture

Improved posture is another long-term benefit of chair yoga. By practicing alignment and body awareness, seniors can benefit from better posture, which helps reduce the risk of musculoskeletal problems.

## 7. Sleep Quality

Chair yoga relaxation techniques can improve sleep quality, helping older people fight sleep disorders or insomnia.

## 8. Enhanced Quality of Life

Finally, chair yoga contributes to a better quality of life for older adults. This allows them to stay active, independent, and connected to their body and mind, promoting a feeling of empowerment and vitality.

# Encouragement to Continue the Practice Beyond 30 Days

Although our chair yoga journey lasts 30 days, the practice is not limited to this period. In fact, chair yoga is great for long-term commitment and incorporating it into your daily routine.

Here's why you should continue practicing chair yoga after the first 30 days:

### 1. Habit Formation

In 30 days, you've probably established a chair yoga routine. Continuing this practice will help cement the habit, ensuring that chair yoga becomes an integral part of your daily life.

### 2. Ongoing Progress

As you've experienced, chair yoga provides a wide range of physical and mental benefits. To reap these rewards consistently, it's crucial to practice regularly and continue building on your progress.

### 3. Health Maintenance

A long-term practice of chair yoga is a proactive approach to maintaining your health and well-being.

This can help prevent age-related problems, such as muscle weakness, joint stiffness, and lack of balance, from becoming significant obstacles.

### 4. Sense of Community

Practicing chair yoga for a long time can also foster a sense of community. Whether you're part of a group class or connecting with other students online, you can share experiences, ideas, and encouragement, creating a supportive environment.

### 5. Emotional and Mental Resilience

Chair yoga's mindfulness and relaxation components provide ongoing support for your emotional and mental well-being. Consistent practice helps you develop the tools to cope with stress, anxiety, and other challenges that life may present.

### 6. Adaptation and Exploration

With time, you'll become more comfortable with chair yoga and can explore more advanced poses and variations. The workout progresses as you go and the journey becomes an exciting exploration of your physical and mental abilities

# Additional Resources for Further Exploration

To dig deeper practicing chair yoga and gaining knowledge, you can explore a variety of resources. Here are some suggestions:

1. **Books:** There are many books available that delve into chair yoga, its history, principles, and detailed instructions. Study titles from renowned authors and yoga experts to increase your understanding of the practice.

You can also check out my other book **(chair yoga for weight loss)** and experience the simple and effortless method to help your weight loss journey.

2. **Online Classes:** Many online platforms offer chair yoga classes and tutorials, making it convenient to practice from the comfort of your own home. Seek out reputable instructors and platforms that cater to seniors.

3. **Local Classes:** If you prefer in-person instruction, explore local community centers, gyms,

or yoga studios that offer chair yoga classes. These courses also often provide opportunities for social engagement.

**4. Apps:** There are mobile apps specifically for chair yoga that provide guided sessions, progress tracking, and reminders to help you maintain your practice.

**5. YouTube Channel:** Many yoga instructors share chair yoga exercises on YouTube. This can be a valuable resource for a variety of practice activities and tutorials.

**6. Community Groups:** Online forums and social media groups focused on chair yoga for seniors can connect you with like-minded people, allowing you to share experiences, book questions, and get support.

**7. Personalized Instruction:** If you're looking for personalized instruction, consider working with a certified chair yoga instructor who can tailor sessions to your needs and your specific goals.

**8. Workshops and Retreats:** Find chair yoga workshops and retreats in your area or online. These events often offer in-depth learning experiences and networking opportunities with other chair yoga enthusiasts.

**9. Meditation and Mindfulness Resources:** Explore mindfulness and meditation practices, complementary to chair yoga, to improve your mental health and emotional resilience.

In conclusion, chair yoga for seniors over 60 is a transformative practice that can significantly improve your physical health, mental clarity, and overall quality of life. Its numerous long-term benefits, including enhanced flexibility, better balance, pain management, and improved mental well-being, make it a valuable addition to your daily routine. We strongly encourage you to continue your chair yoga practice beyond the initial 30 days, as it offers ongoing physical and emotional benefits. Whether you explore additional resources, engage with a community, or deepen your understanding of the practice, chair yoga has the potential to become a lifelong companion on your journey to health and wellness.